CENTERS FOR MEDICARE & MEDICAID SERVICES

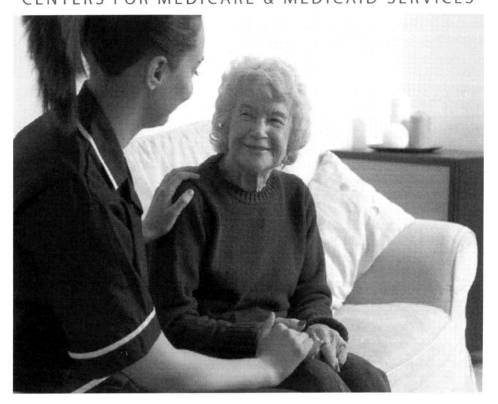

Medicare and Home Health Care

This is the official U.S. government booklet about Medicare home health care benefits for people with Original Medicare. This booklet has important information about the following:

- Who is eligible
- What services are covered
- How to find and compare home health agencies
- Your Medicare rights

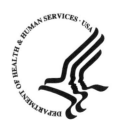

The information in this booklet was correct when it was printed. Changes may occur after printing. Call 1-800-MEDICARE (1-800-633-4227), or visit www.medicare.gov to get the most current information. TTY users should call 1-877-486-2048.

"Medicare and Home Health Care" isn't a legal document. Official Medicare Program legal guidance is contained in the relevant statutes, regulations, and rulings.

Table of Contents

Introduction 4

Section 1: Medicare Coverage of Home Health Care 5
Who's eligible? 5
Eligibility is also based on the amount of services you need 6
How Medicare pays for home health care 7
What Medicare covers 8
What isn't covered? 10
What you have to pay 10
Home Health Advance Beneficiary Notice 11
Your right to a fast appeal 12
General Medicare appeal rights 14

Section 2: Choosing a Home Health Agency 15
Finding a Medicare-certified home health agency 15
Comparing home health agencies 15
Comparing quality 16
Home Health Agency Checklist 17
Special rules for home health care 18
Find out more about home health agencies 18

Section 3: Getting Home Health Care 19
Your plan of care 19
Your rights as a person with Medicare 20
Where to file a complaint about the quality of your home health care 21
Home Health Care Checklist 22

Section 4: Getting the Help You Need 23
Extra Help paying for Medicare Prescription Drug Coverage (Part D) . . 23
State Pharmacy Assistance Programs (SPAPs) 24
Medicaid 24
Medicare Savings Programs (Help with Medicare costs) 25
For more information 25
Help with questions about home health coverage 26
What you need to know about fraud 27

Definitions 29

Index 31

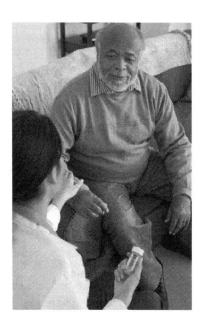

Introduction

Many health care treatments that were once offered only in a hospital or a doctor's office can now be done in your home. Home health care is usually less expensive, more convenient, and just as effective as care you get in a hospital or skilled nursing facility. In general, the goal of home health care is to provide treatment for an illness or injury. Home health care helps you get better, regain your independence, and become as self-sufficient as possible.

Medicare pays for you to get certain health care services in your home if you meet certain eligibility criteria and if the services are considered reasonable and necessary for the treatment of your illness or injury. This is known as the Medicare home health benefit.

If you get your Medicare benefits through a Medicare health plan (not Original Medicare) check your plan's membership materials, and contact the plan for details about how the plan provides your Medicare-covered home health benefits.

Section 1:
Medicare Coverage of Home Health Care

Who's eligible?

If you have Medicare, you can use your home health benefits if you meet all the following conditions:

1. You must be under the care of a doctor, and you must be getting services under a plan of care established and reviewed regularly by a doctor.
2. You must need, and a doctor must certify that you need, one or more of the following.
    - Intermittent skilled nursing care
    - Physical therapy
    - Speech-language pathology services
    - Continued occupational therapy

    See page 8 for more detail on these services.
3. The home health agency caring for you must be approved by Medicare (Medicare-certified).
4. You must be homebound, and a doctor must certify that you're homebound. To be homebound means the following:
    - Leaving your home isn't recommended because of your condition.
    - Your condition keeps you from leaving home without help (such as using a wheelchair or walker, needing special transportation, or getting help from another person).
    - Leaving home takes a considerable and taxing effort.

A person may leave home for medical treatment or short, infrequent absences for non-medical reasons, such as attending religious services. You can still get home health care if you attend adult day care, but you would get the home care services in your home.

Words in red are defined on pages 29–30.

Eligibility is also based on the amount of services you need

If you meet the conditions above, Medicare pays for your covered home health services for as long as you're eligible and your doctor certifies you need them. If you need more than part-time or "intermittent" skilled nursing care, you aren't eligible for the home health benefit.

To decide whether you're eligible for home health care, Medicare defines part-time or "intermittent" as skilled nursing care that's needed or given on fewer than 7 days each week or less than 8 hours each day over a period of 21 days (or less) with some exceptions in special circumstances.

Hour and day limits may be extended in exceptional circumstances when your doctor can predict when your need for care will end.

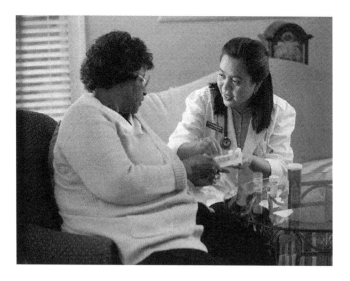

How Medicare pays for home health care

In Original Medicare, Medicare pays your Medicare-certified home health agency one payment for covered services you get during a 60-day period. This 60-day period is called an "episode of care." The payment is based on your condition and care needs.

Getting treatment from a home health agency that's Medicare-certified can reduce your out-of-pocket costs. A Medicare-certified home health agency agrees to the following conditions:

- To be paid by Medicare
- To accept only the amount Medicare approves for their services

Medicare's home health benefit only pays for services provided by the home health agency. Other medical services, such as visits to your doctor, are generally still covered by your other Medicare benefits. Look in your copy of the "Medicare & You" handbook, mailed to each Medicare household every fall, for information on how these services are covered under Medicare. To view or print this booklet, visit http://go.usa.gov/iDJ. You can also call 1-800-MEDICARE (1-800-633-4227) if you have questions about your Medicare benefits. TTY users should call 1-877-486-2048.

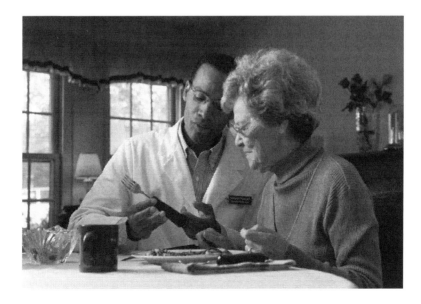

What Medicare covers

If you're eligible for Medicare-covered home health care (see page 5), Medicare covers the following services if they're reasonable and necessary for the treatment of your illness or injury:

- **Skilled nursing care.** Skilled nursing services are covered when they're given on a part-time or intermittent basis. In order for skilled nursing care to be covered by the Medicare home health benefit, your care must be necessary and ordered by your doctor for your specific condition. You must **not** need full time nursing care and you must be homebound. See page 5.

  Skilled nursing services are given by either a registered nurse (RN) or a licensed practical nurse (LPN). If you get services from a LPN, your care will be supervised by a RN. Home health nurses provide direct care and teach you and your caregivers about your care. They also manage, observe, and evaluate your care. Examples of skilled nursing care include: giving IV drugs, shots, or tube feedings; changing dressings; and teaching about prescription drugs or diabetes care. Any service that could be done safely by a non-medical person (or by yourself) without the supervision of a nurse, **isn't** skilled nursing care.

  Home health aide services may be covered when given on a part-time or intermittent basis if needed as support services for skilled nursing care. Home health aide services must be part of the care for your illness or injury. Medicare doesn't cover home health aide services unless you're also getting skilled care such as nursing care or other physical therapy, occupational therapy, or speech-language pathology services from the home health agency.

- **Physical therapy, occupational therapy, and speech-language pathology services.** Medicare uses the following criteria to assess whether these therapy services are reasonable and necessary in the home setting:

    1. The therapy services must be a specific, safe, and effective treatment for your condition.
    2. The therapy services must be complex or your condition must require services that can safely and effectively be performed only by qualified therapists.

3. One of the three following conditions must exist:
   - It's expected that your condition will improve in a reasonable and generally-predictable period of time.
   - Your condition requires a skilled therapist to safely and effectively establish a maintenance program.
   - Your condition requires a skilled therapist to safely and effectively perform maintenance therapy.
4. The amount, frequency, and duration of the services must be reasonable.

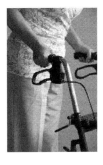

- **Medical social services.** These services are covered when given under the direction of a doctor to help you with social and emotional concerns related to your illness. This might include counseling or help finding resources in your community.
- **Medical supplies.** Supplies, like wound dressings, are covered when they are ordered as part of your care.

Durable medical equipment, when ordered by a doctor, is paid separately by Medicare. This equipment must meet certain criteria to be covered. Medicare usually pays 80% of the Medicare-approved amount for certain pieces of medical equipment, such as a wheelchair or walker. If your home health agency doesn't supply durable medical equipment directly, the home health agency staff will usually arrange for a home equipment supplier to bring the items you need to your home.

Note: Before your home health care begins, the home health agency should tell you how much of your bill Medicare will pay. The agency should also tell you if any items or services they give you aren't covered by Medicare, and how much you will have to pay for them. This should be explained by both talking with you and in writing.

Note: The home health agency is responsible for meeting **all** your medical, nursing, rehabilitative, social, and discharge planning needs, as reflected in your home health plan of care. See page 19. This includes skilled therapy services for a condition that may not be the primary reason for getting home health services. Home health agencies are required to perform a comprehensive assessment of each of your care needs when you're admitted to the home health agency, and communicate those needs to the doctor responsible for the plan of care. After that, home health agencies are required to routinely assess your needs.

What isn't covered?

Below are some examples of what Medicare doesn't pay for:

- 24-hour-a-day care at home.
- Meals delivered to your home.
- Homemaker services like shopping, cleaning, and laundry when this is the only care you need, and when these services aren't related to your plan of care. See page 19.
- Personal care given by home health aides like bathing, dressing, and using the bathroom when this is the only care you need.

Talk to your doctor or the home health agency if you have questions about whether certain services are covered. You can also call 1-800-MEDICARE (1-800-633-4227). TTY users should call 1-877-486-2048.

Note: If you have a Medigap (Medicare Supplement Insurance) policy or other health insurance coverage, be sure to tell your doctor or other health care provider so your bills get paid correctly.

What you have to pay

You may be billed for the following:

- Medical services and supplies that Medicare doesn't pay for when you agree to pay out of pocket for them. The home health agency should give you a notice called the Home Health Advance Beneficiary Notice (HHABN) before giving you services and supplies that Medicare doesn't cover. See page 11.
- 20% of the Medicare-approved amount for Medicare-covered medical equipment such as wheelchairs, walkers, and oxygen equipment.

Home Health Advance Beneficiary Notice

The home health agency should give you a written notice called a Home Health Advance Beneficiary Notice (HHABN) in the following situations:

- The home health agency reduces or stops providing you with some home health services or supplies for business-related reasons while continuing other home health services.
- The home health agency reduces or stops providing home health services or supplies because your doctor has changed your orders.
- The home health agency plans to give you a home health service or supply that Medicare probably won't pay for.

If a home health agency reduces or stops providing certain services or supplies, you may have the option to keep getting them. The HHABN will explain what service or supply is going to be reduced or stopped and give you instructions on what you can do if you want to keep getting the service or supply.

When you get an HHABN because Medicare isn't expected to pay for a medical service or supply, the notice should describe the service and/or supply, and explain why Medicare probably won't pay.

The HHABN gives clear directions for getting an official decision from Medicare about payment for home health services and supplies and for filing an appeal if Medicare won't pay.

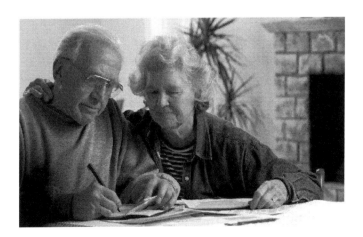

Home Health Advance Beneficiary Notice (continued)

In general, to get an official decision on payment, you should do the following:

- Keep getting the home health services and/or supplies if you think you need them. The home health agency must tell you how much they will cost. Talk to your doctor and family about this decision.
- Understand you may have to pay the home health agency for these services and/or supplies.
- Ask the home health agency to send your claim to Medicare so that Medicare will make a decision about payment. You have the right to have the agency bill Medicare for your care.

If Original Medicare pays for your care, you will get back all of your payments, except for any applicable coinsurance or deductibles, including any coinsurance payments you made for durable medical equipment.

Your right to a fast appeal

When all your covered home health services are ending, you may have the right to a fast appeal if you think these services are ending too soon. During a fast appeal, an independent reviewer called a Quality Improvement Organization (QIO) looks at your case and decides if you need home health services to continue. The QIO is a group of practicing doctors and other health care experts paid by the Federal government to check and improve the care given to Medicare patients.

Your home health agency will give you a written notice called the Notice of Medicare Provider Non-Coverage at least 2 days before all covered services end. If you don't get this notice, ask for it. Read the notice carefully. It contains the following information:

- The date all your covered services will end
- How to ask for a fast appeal
- Your right to get a detailed notice about why your services are ending

If you ask for a fast appeal, the Quality Improvement Organization (QIO) will ask for your opinion about why you believe coverage of your home health services should continue. The QIO will also look at your medical information and talk to your doctor. The QIO will notify you of its decision as soon as possible, generally no later than 2 days after the effective date of the Notice of Medicare Provider Non-Coverage.

If the QIO decides your home health services should continue, Medicare may continue to cover your home health care services except for any applicable coinsurance or deductibles.

If the QIO decides that your coverage should end, you will have to pay for any services you got after the date on the Notice of Medicare Provider Non-Coverage that says your covered services should end. You won't be responsible for paying for any covered services provided before that date.

You may stop getting services on or before the date given on the Notice of Medicare Provider Non-Coverage and avoid paying for any further services. Before giving you services that Medicare may not pay for, your home health agency should give you a Home Health Advance Beneficiary Notice (HHABN) with an estimate of how much these services will cost.

General Medicare appeal rights

After Medicare makes a decision on a claim, you have the right to a fair, efficient, and timely process for appealing health care payment decisions or initial determinations on items or services you got.

You may appeal if either of the following is true:
- A service or item you got isn't covered, and you think it should be.
- A service or item is denied, and you think it should be paid.

The company that handles claims for Medicare will send you a list of your claims, called The Medicare Summary Notice (MSN), every 3 months. This notice tells you if your claim is approved or denied. If the claim is denied, the reason for the denial will be included on the notice. The notice will also include information about how to file an appeal. Review this notice carefully, and follow the instructions to file an appeal.

You can file an appeal if you disagree with Medicare's decision on payment or coverage for the items or services you got. If you appeal, ask your doctor, health care provider, or supplier for any information that might help your case. You should keep a copy of everything you send to Medicare as part of your appeal.

For more information on your right to a fast appeal and other Medicare appeal rights, look at your "Medicare & You" handbook or "Your Medicare Rights and Protections" booklet. To view or print this booklet, visit http://go.usa.gov/low. You can also call 1-800-MEDICARE (1-800-633-4227). TTY users should call 1-877-486-2048.

Section 2: Choosing a Home Health Agency

Finding a Medicare-certified home health agency

If your doctor decides you need home health care, you may choose an agency from the participating Medicare-certified home health agencies that serve your area. Home health agencies are certified to make sure they meet certain Federal health and safety requirements. Your choice should be honored by your doctor, hospital discharge planner, or other referring agency. You have a say in which agency you use, but your choices may be limited by agency availability, or by your insurance coverage. (Medicare Advantage Plans or other Medicare health plans may require that you get home health services from agencies they contract with.)

Comparing home health agencies

Use Medicare's "Home Health Compare" web tool by visiting www.medicare.gov/HHCompare to compare home health agencies in your area. You can compare home health agencies by the types of services they offer and the quality of care they provide. Home Health Compare provides the following information about home health agencies:

- Name, address, and telephone number
- Services offered (such as nursing care, physical therapy, occupational therapy, speech-language pathology services, medical/social services, and home health aide services)
- Initial date of Medicare certification
- Type of ownership (For Profit, Government, Non-Profit)
- Information about the quality of care provided (quality measures)

Words in red are defined on pages 29–30.

Comparing quality

Some home health agencies do a better job of caring for their patients than others. Home health agencies give quality care when they give their patients care and treatment known to get the best results for each patient's condition. Use Home Health Compare to see how well home health agencies in your area care for their patients. You can compare agencies based on various measures of quality and against state and national averages.

Here's an example of the information you'll find on Home Health Compare:

Quality Measures	Percentage for XYZ Home Care Agency	State Average	National Average
HIGHER PERCENTAGES ARE BETTER			
Percentage of patients who get better at walking or moving around	71%	76%	82%
Percentage of patients who get better at getting in and out of bed	74%	72%	72%
Percentage of patients who have less pain when moving around	59%	80%	76%
Percentage of patients whose wounds improved or healed after an operation	77%	76%	80%

Home Health Agency Checklist

Use this checklist when choosing a home health agency.

Name of the Home Health Agency_____

Question	Yes	No	Comments
1. Medicare-certified?			
2. Medicaid-certified (if you have both Medicare and Medicaid)?			
3. Offers the specific health care services I need (like skilled nursing services or physical therapy)?			
4. Meets my special needs (like language or cultural preferences)?			
5. Offers the personal care services I need (like help bathing, dressing, and using the bathroom)?			
6. Offers the support services I need, or can help me arrange for additional services, such as Meals on Wheels, that I may need?			
7. Has staff that can provide the type and hours of care my doctor ordered and start when I need them?			
8. Is recommended by my hospital discharge planner, doctor, or social worker?			
9. Has staff available at night and on weekends for emergencies?			
10. Explained what my insurance will cover and what I must pay out-of-pocket?			
11. Does background checks on all staff?			
12. Has letters from satisfied patients, family members, and doctors that testify to the home health agency providing good care?			

Special rules for home health care

In general, most Medicare-certified home health agencies will accept all Medicare patients. An agency isn't required to accept a patient if it can't meet the patient's medical needs. An agency shouldn't refuse to take a specific Medicare patient because of the patient's condition, unless the agency would also refuse to take other patients with the same condition.

Medicare will only pay for you to get care from one home health agency at a time. You may decide to end your relationship with one agency and choose another at any time. Contact your doctor to get a referral to a new agency. You should tell both the agency you're leaving and the new agency you choose that you're changing home health agencies.

Find out more about home health agencies

Your State Survey Agency, the agency that inspects and certifies home health agencies for Medicare, also has information about home health agencies. Ask them for the state survey report on the home health agency of interest to you. Call 1-800-MEDICARE (1-800-633-4227) to get your State Survey Agency's telephone number. TTY users should call 1-877-486-2048. You can also visit www.medicare.gov.

In some cases, your local long-term care ombudsman may have information on the home health agencies in your area. Visit www.ltcombudsman.org. You can also call the Eldercare Locator at 1-800-677-1116, or visit www.eldercare.gov.

To find out more about home health agencies, you can do any of the following:

- Ask your doctor, hospital discharge planner, or social worker. Or, ask friends or family about their home health care experiences.
- Use a senior community referral service, or other community agencies that help you with your health care.
- Look in your telephone directory in the Yellow Pages under "home care" or "home health care."

Section 3: Getting Home Health Care

Usually, once your doctor refers you for home health services, staff from the home health agency will come to your home to talk to you about your needs and ask you some questions about your health. The home health agency will also talk to your doctor about your care and keep your doctor updated about your progress. Doctor's orders are needed to start care.

Your plan of care

Your home health agency will work with you and your doctor to develop your plan of care. A plan of care lists what kind of services and care you should get for your health problem. You have the right to be involved in any decisions about your Your plan of care includes the following:

- What services you need
- Which health care professionals should give these services
- How often you will need the services
- The medical equipment you need
- What results your doctor expects from your treatment

Your home health agency must provide you with all the home care listed in your plan of care, including services and medical supplies. The agency may do this through its own staff or through an arrangement with another agency; or by hiring nurses, therapists, home health aides, and medical social service counselors to meet your needs.

Words in red are defined on pages 29–30.

Your plan of care (continued)

Your doctor and home health team review your plan of care as often as necessary, but at least once every 60 days. If your health problems change, the home health team should tell your doctor right away. Your plan of care will be reviewed and may change. Your home health team should only change your plan of care with your doctor's approval. Your home health team should also tell you about any changes in your plan of care. If you have a question about your care, or if you feel your needs aren't being met, talk to both your doctor and the home health team.

The home health team will teach you (and your family or friends who are helping you) to continue any care you may need, including wound care, therapy, and disease management. You should learn to recognize problems like infection or shortness of breath, and know what to do or whom to contact if they happen.

Your rights as a person with Medicare

In general, as a person with Medicare getting home health care from a Medicare-certified home health agency, you're guaranteed certain rights, including the following:

- To get a written notice of your rights before your care starts
- To have your home and property treated with respect
- To be told, in advance, what care you will be getting and when your plan of care is going to change
- To participate in your care planning and treatment
- To get written information about your privacy rights and your appeal rights
- To have your personal information kept private
- To get written and verbal information about how much Medicare is expected to pay and how much you will have to pay for any services that you will be getting
- To make complaints about your care and have the home health agency follow up on them
- To know the phone number of the home-health hotline in your state where you can call with complaints or questions about your care

Read more about these rights and protections in the following publications:

- "Your Medicare Rights and Protections"—Visit http://go.usa.gov/low.
- "Medicare & You" handbook—Visit http://go.usa.gov/iDJ.

You can also call 1-800-MEDICARE (1-800-633-4227). TTY users should call 1-877-486-2048.

Where to file a complaint about the quality of your home health care

If you have a complaint about the quality of care you're getting from a home health agency, you should call either of the following organizations:

- Your state home health hotline. Your home health agency should give you this number when you start getting home health services.
- The Quality Improvement Organization (QIO) in your state. The QIO is a group of practicing doctors and other health care experts paid by the Federal government to check and improve the care given to Medicare patients. To get the telephone number for your QIO, visit www.medicare.gov. You can also call 1-800-MEDICARE.

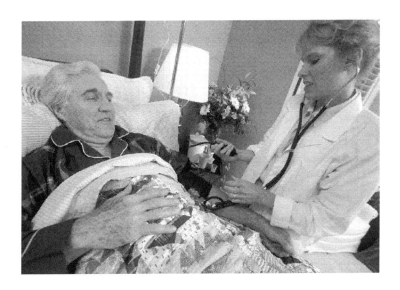

Home Health Care Checklist

This checklist can help you (and your family or friends who are helping you) monitor your home health care. Use this checklist to help ensure that you're getting good quality home health care.

When I get my home health care	Yes	No	Comments
1. The staff is polite and treats me and my family with respect.			
2. The staff explains my plan of care to me and my family, lets us participate in creating the plan of care, and lets us know ahead of time of any changes.			
3. The staff is properly trained and licensed to perform the type of health care I need.			
4. The agency explains what to do if I have a problem with the staff or the care I'm getting.			
5. The agency responds quickly to my requests.			
6. The staff checks my physical and emotional condition at each visit.			
7. The staff responds quickly to changes in my health or behavior.			
8. The staff checks my home and suggests changes to meet my special needs and to ensure my safety.			
9. The staff has told me what to do if I have an emergency.			
10. The agency and its staff protect my privacy.			

Section 4: Getting the Help You Need

Extra Help paying for Medicare Prescription Drug Coverage (Part D)

You may qualify for Extra Help, also called the low-income subsidy (LIS), from Medicare to pay prescription drug costs if your yearly income and resources are below the following limits in 2010:

- Single person—Income less than $16,245 and resources less than $12,510
- Married person living with a spouse—Income less than $21,855 and resources less than $25,010

These amounts may change in 2011. You may qualify even if you have a higher income (like if you still work, or if you live in Alaska or Hawaii, or have dependents living with you). Resources include money in a checking or savings account, stocks, and bonds. Resources **don't** include your home, car, household items, burial plot, up to $1,500 for burial expenses (per person), or life insurance policies. For more information, call Social Security at 1-800-772-1213, or visit www.socialsecurity.gov. TTY users should call 1-800-325-0778. All information you share is confidential.

Words in red are defined on pages 29–30.

State Pharmacy Assistance Programs (SPAPs)

Many states have State Pharmacy Assistance Programs (SPAPs) that help certain people pay for prescription drugs based on financial need, age, or medical condition. Each SPAP makes its own rules about how to provide drug coverage to its members. Depending on your state, the SPAP will help you in different ways. To find out about the SPAP in your state, call your State Health Insurance Assistance Program (SHIP). To get their number, visit www.medicare.gov or call 1-800-MEDICARE (1-800-633-4227). TTY users should call 1-877-486-2048.

Medicaid

Medicaid is a joint Federal and state program that helps pay medical costs if you have limited income and resources and meet other requirements. Some people qualify for both Medicare and Medicaid (these people are called "dual eligibles").

- If you have Medicare and full Medicaid coverage, most of your health care costs are covered.
- Medicaid programs vary by state. They may also be called by different names, like "Medical Assistance" or "Medi-Cal."
- People with Medicaid may get coverage for services that Medicare doesn't fully cover, such as nursing home and home health care.
- Each state has different Medicaid income and resource limits and other eligibility requirements.
- In some states, you may need to apply for Medicare to be eligible for Medicaid.
- Call your State Medical Assistance (Medicaid) office for more information and to see if you qualify. Call 1-800-MEDICARE, and say "Medicaid" to get the telephone number for your State Medical Assistance (Medicaid) office. You can also visit www.medicare.gov.

Medicare Savings Programs (Help with Medicare costs)

States have programs that pay Medicare premiums and, in some cases, may also pay your Part A (Hospital Insurance) and Part B (Medical Insurance) deductibles and coinsurance. These programs help people with Medicare save money each year.

To qualify for a Medicare Savings Program, you must meet all of these conditions:

- Have Part A
- Single person—Have monthly income less than $1,239 and resources less than $8,100
- Married and living with a spouse—Have monthly income less than $1,660 and resources less than $12,910

Note: These amounts may change each year. Many states figure your income and resources differently or may not have limits at all, so you may qualify in your state even if your income is higher. Resources include money in a checking or savings account, stocks, and bonds. Resources don't include your home, car, burial plot, up to $1,500 for burial expenses (per person), furniture, or other household items.

For more information

- Call or visit your State Medical Assistance (Medicaid) office, and ask for information on Medicare Savings Programs. The names of these programs and how they work may vary by state. Call if you think you qualify for any of these programs, even if you aren't sure.
- Call 1-800-MEDICARE (1-800-633-4227), and say "Medicaid" to get the telephone number for your state. TTY users should call 1-877-486-2048.
- Visit http://go.usa.gov/loA to view the brochure, "Get Help With Your Medicare Costs: Getting Started."
- Contact your State Health Insurance Assistance Program (SHIP) for free health insurance counseling. To get their number, call 1-800-MEDICARE. You can also visit www.medicare.gov, and under "Help & Support" select "Useful Phone Numbers and Websites." Then, search by the word "organization" or "SHIP."

Help with questions about home health coverage

If you have questions about your Medicare home health care benefits or coverage and you're in Original Medicare, call 1-800-MEDICARE (1-800-633-4227). TTY users should call 1-877-486-2048. If you get your Medicare benefits through a Medicare health plan, call your plan.

You may also call the State Health Insurance Assistance Program (SHIP). Every State and territory, plus Puerto Rico, the Virgin Islands, and the District of Columbia has a SHIP with counselors who can give you free health insurance information and help. The SHIP counselors answer questions about Medicare's home health benefits and what Medicare, Medicaid, and other types of insurance pay for. In addition, these counselors help with the following:

- Medicare payment questions.
- Questions about buying a Medigap (Medicare Supplement Insurance) policy or long-term care insurance.
- Concerns about payment denials and appeals.
- Medicare rights and protections.
- Complaints about your care or treatment.
- Choosing a Medicare health plan.

To get the telephone number for your SHIP, visit www.medicare.gov on the web, or call 1-800-MEDICARE.

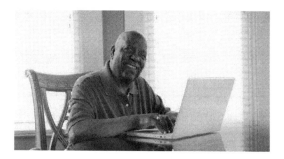

What you need to know about fraud

In general, most home health agencies are honest and use correct billing information. Unfortunately, there may be some who commit fraud. Fraud wastes Medicare dollars and takes money that could be used to pay claims. You're important in the fight to prevent fraud, waste, and abuse in the Medicare Program.

You should look for the following:

- Home health visits that your doctor ordered, but that you didn't get.
- Visits by home health staff that you didn't request and that you don't need.
- Bills for services and equipment you never got.
- Fake signatures (yours or your doctor's) on medical forms or equipment orders.
- Pressure to accept items and services that you don't need or that Medicare doesn't cover.
- Items listed on your Medicare Summary Notice that you don't think you got or used.
- Home health services your doctor didn't order. The doctor who approves home health services for you should know you, and should be involved in your care. If your plan of care changes, make sure that your doctor was involved in making those changes.
- A home health agency that offers you free goods or services in exchange for your Medicare number. Treat your Medicare card like a credit card or cash. Never give your Medicare or Medicaid number to people who tell you a service is free, and they need your number for their records.

The best way to protect your home health benefit is to know what Medicare covers and to know what your doctor has planned for you. If you don't understand something in your plan of care, ask questions.

Reporting fraud

If you suspect fraud, here's what you can do:

- Contact your home health agency to be sure the bill is correct.

- Call the Office of Inspector General Hotline:
    By Phone: 1-800-HHS-TIPS (1-800-447-8477)
    By Fax: 1-800-223-2164 (no more than 10 pages)
    By E-Mail: HHSTips@oig.hhs.gov
    By Mail: Office of the Inspector General
    HHS TIPS Hotline
    P.O. Box 23489
    Washington, DC 20026

    Please note that it is current Hotline policy not to respond directly to written communications.

- If you live in Florida, call Medicare's Florida Fraud Hotline:
    By Phone: 1-866-417-2078
    By E-Mail: floridamedicarefraud@hp.com

- Call 1-800-MEDICARE (1-800-633-4227). TTY users should call 1-877-486-2048.

Important: If you're reporting a possible case of Medicare fraud, please provide as much identifying information as possible. Include the person or company's name, address, and phone number. Details should include the basics of who, what, when, where, why, and how.

Definitions

Appeal—An appeal is the action you can take if you disagree with a coverage or payment decision made by Medicare, your Medicare health plan, or your Medicare Prescription Drug Plan. You can appeal if Medicare or your plan denies one of the following:

- Your request for a health care service, supply, or prescription that you think you should be able to get
- Your request for payment for health care or a prescription drug you already got
- Your request to change the amount you must pay for a prescription drug

You can also appeal if you are already getting coverage and Medicare or your plan stops paying.

Durable Medical Equipment—Certain medical equipment, such as a walker, wheelchair, or hospital bed, that is ordered by your doctor for use in the home.

Medicaid—A joint Federal and state program that helps with medical costs for some people with limited income and resources. Medicaid programs vary from state to state, but most health care costs are covered if you qualify for both Medicare and Medicaid.

Medicare Advantage Plan (Part C)—A type of Medicare health plan offered by a private company that contracts with Medicare to provide you with all your Medicare Part A and Part B benefits. Medicare Advantage Plans include Health Maintenance Organizations, Preferred Provider Organizations, Private Fee-for-Service Plans, Special Needs Plans, and Medicare Medical Savings Account Plans. If you're enrolled in a Medicare Advantage Plan, Medicare services are covered through the plan and aren't paid for under Original Medicare. Most Medicare Advantage Plans offer prescription drug coverage.

Medicare Health Plan—A plan offered by a private company that contracts with Medicare to provide Part A and Part B benefits to people with Medicare who enroll in the plan.

Medigap Policy—Medicare Supplement Insurance sold by private insurance companies to fill "gaps" in Original Medicare coverage.

Original Medicare—Original Medicare is fee-for-service coverage under which the government pays your health care providers directly for your Part A and/or Part B benefits.

State Health Insurance Assistance Program (SHIP)—A state program that gets money from the Federal government to give free local health insurance counseling to people with Medicare.

Index

A
Appeal 11–14, 29

C
Complaint 21

D
Durable Medical Equipment 9, 29

E
Eldercare Locator 18
Eligibility 5–6
Episode of Care 7

F
Fraud 27–28

H
Homebound 5
Home Health Advance Beneficiary Notice (HHABN) 11–12
Home Health Agency 15
Home Health Compare 15

L
Long-term Care Ombudsman 18

M
Medicaid 24, 25, 29
Medical Social Services 9
Medical Supplies 9
Medicare Advantage Plan 15, 29
Medicare-approved Amount 9, 10
Medicare Health Plan 4, 15, 26, 30
Medigap (Medicare Supplement Insurance) Policy 26, 30

O
Occupational Therapy 5, 8
Official Decision 12
Original Medicare 4, 26, 30

P
Payment 26
Physical Therapy 5, 8
Plan of Care 5, 9, 19, 20
Prescription Drugs 23

Q
Quality 15–16
Quality Improvement Organization (QIO) 12–13

S
Skilled Nursing Care 5, 8
Speech-Language Pathology Services 5, 8
State Health Insurance Assistance Program (SHIP) 25, 30
State Survey Agency 18

Made in the USA
Middletown, DE
08 October 2015